I0006489

Dissertation Discovery Company and University of Florida are dedicated to making scholarly works more discoverable and accessible throughout the world.

This dissertation, "Data Acquistition of Fast Rise Time Pulses of Magnetic Thin Films" by Peter Tappen Fairchild, was obtained from University of Florida and is being sold with permission from the author. The content of this dissertation has not been altered in any way. We have altered the formatting in order to facilitate the ease of printing and reading of the dissertation.

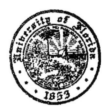

DEDICATION

This work is dedicated to all those who
have helped me along the way.

ACKNOWLEDGEMENTS

The author wishes to express sincere appreciation to his committee members, Dr. J. K. Watson, Dr. A. J. Brodersen and Dr. A. H. Paige for their guidance and encouragement throughout the preparation of this thesis. The author is also grateful to Mr. Steve Barnet of Datacom, Inc. who provided much useful technical information concerning the Datacom 8015 data acquisition system.

Special thanks are also owed Messrs. Richard F. Motta and James E. Smith for patiently reviewing the manuscript and to Mrs. Roswitha Zamorano who typed the many drafts.

TABLE OF CONTENTS

LIST OF TABLES

LIST OF FIGURES

Abstract of Thesis Presented to the Graduate Council·
of the University of Florida in Partial Fulfillment of the Requirements
for the Degree of Master of Engineering

DATA ACQUISITION OF FAST RISE TIME
PULSES OF MAGNETIC THIN FILMS

By

Peter Tappen Fairchild

June, 1973

Chairman: Dr. J. K. Watson
Major Department: Electrical Engineering

The development of an instrument system capable of measuring very

fast rise time pulses and storing digitized data for subsequent

computer analysis is described. The system is comprised of a sampling

oscilloscope (input), a data acquisition system (storage and data

output), and associated FORTRAN software.

The sampling capability of the Tektronix 661 sampling oscilloscope

and the digitizing and storage capability of Datacom's 8015 data acquisi-

tion system (DAS) are used to best advantage. The method used to inter-

face these two pieces of commercial equipment and the provision of soft-

ware support are the focus of attention.

The Tektronix 661 sampling oscilloscope vertical and horizontal control

voltages are transformed to logic signals capable of controlling the DAS.

The vertical deflection voltage is scaled to the DAS full scale ($\pm 10V$) input.

The DAS uses magnetic tape as an output medium. The FORTRAN software

package reads the tape, reconstructs the signal, plots the waveform,

integrates the area under the curve and calculates the switching time.

The system will be utilized in characterizing the switching properties

of magnetic thin films.

INTRODUCTION

This thesis describes the development of a data acquisition and processing system for measuring and analyzing
fast rise time pulses.

Advantage is taken of the sampling capability of the
Tektronix 661 sampling oscilloscope, which can measure fast
rise time pulses. A Datacom 8015 data acquisition system
provided a storage facility and a data transfer media
(magnetic tape). Referring to Fig. I.1, we see two problems
are critical in the system development. One of the problems
is interfacing the sampling oscilloscope with the data
acquisition system. The other comes about in reading the
data written on magnetic tape and reducing the data to a
form suitable for interpretation by the experimenter. The
system is to be used to reduce data from research on the
switching characteristics of magnetic thin films. The
important parameters are switching time and the area under
the switching curve. A plot of the waveform is also provided.
The large quantity of data expected in these experiments
made necessary the approach which couples the sampling oscilloscope to the computer. The nanosecond switching speed and
the slow pulse repetition rate posed particular problems in
the design of the interface hardware.

1

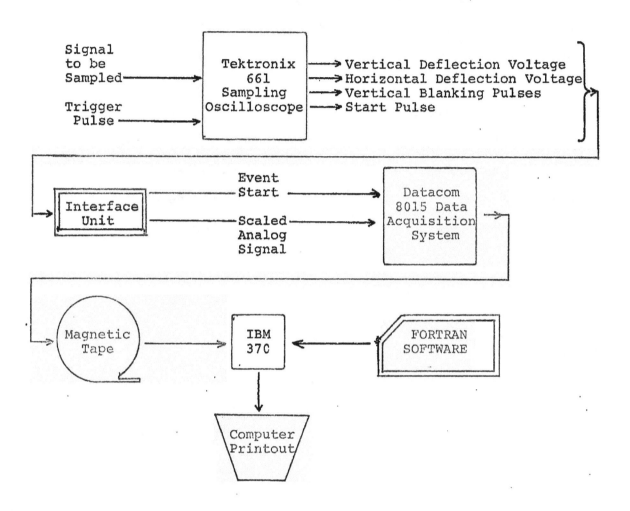

Fig. I.1 Block diagram for the data acquisition system
for fast rise time pulses.

The thesis has five chapters. Chapter I discusses the sampling oscilloscope and the data acquisition system with particular emphasis on the problems of interfacing the two instruments. Chapter II describes the interface hardware in detail. Chapter III discusses the development of the FORTRAN software and describes the program. Chapter IV presents a brief user's manual. There are many ways that the system can be used and this thesis is concerned with one mode of operation. Chapter V summarizes the development effort and the accomplishments of this thesis.

CHAPTER I

COMMERCIAL HARDWARE

In this chapter, the reader will be familiarized with
the commercial equipment used in the fast rise time pulse
data acquisition system. There are two commercial instruments interconnected in this system: 1) the Tektronix 661
sampling oscilloscope; and 2) the Datacom 8015 data acquisition system. Sufficient background information is presented
to enable the reader to understand how and why certain func-
tions are performed in the interface hardware.

The Tektronix 661 sampling oscilloscope is an instrument
that can sample a waveform and display it at a delayed rate.[1]
The sampling oscilloscope accomplishes this by repetitively
sampling a waveform, each sample being taken at a slightly
later point in time. A typical waveform and the samples
taken from it are shown in Fig. 1.1.

The sampling oscilloscope displays the sampled waveform
as a series of dots, each dot representing one sample. The

_____

[1] The concept of "delayed rate" can be illustrated in the
following way. Consider the display of a pulse from a peri-
odic pulse train. The display is actually the composite
of samples of a number of identical pulses in the train.
Thus the rate at which the display is generated on the
oscilloscope CRT is equal to the repetition rate of the
pulse train.

(a)

(b)

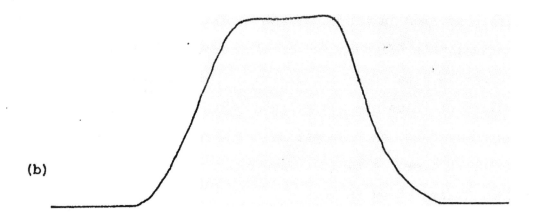

Fig. 1.1   (a) Dots representing the samples taken on
           the waveform; (b) the waveform being sampled,
           which is repeated n times. The input signal
           must have occurred n times since one sample
           is taken per occurrence.

number of samples taken on a waveform can be controlled by the samples/cm setting. Since the real time between each sample is constant, the more samples taken, the longer it takes to display a complete waveform. Since the waveform display is made up of a sequence of dots, the advantage of more samples/cm is that a more continuous display on the screen will be observed.

The vertical position of a dot on the screen is controlled by a deflection voltage on the vertical deflection plates of the cathode ray tube (CRT). The horizontal position of a dot is controlled by a deflection voltage on the horizontal deflection plates of the CRT. The dot is formed by an electron beam which illuminates the phosphor screen. The beam is turned on and off to form the dots by a vertical blanking pulse. These three voltages, the vertical deflection voltage, the horizontal deflection voltage and the vertical blanking pulses provide necessary input signals to the interface. The interfacing problem consists basically of transferring one sweep of the sampling oscilloscope into the Datacom 8015 data acquisition system (DAS).

A sweep is the movement of the electron beam across the screen from the viewer's left to right. The beam vertical movement is controlled by a voltage which is proportional to the sample taken at that instant. The horizontal movement is controlled by a voltage which is an inverted ramp. These two voltages are available to the user as front panel connections. The vertical blanking pulse is a pulse which

occurs each time a sample is taken. The interface unit
modifies these sweep control voltages to drive the data
acquisition system (DAS).

The DAS is a system which transforms analog voltage
data to digital data on magnetic tape. The DAS can multi-
plex up to 16 analog inputs (which have a full scale limit
of ±10V), digitize the analog signal, store the data in a 1K
memory, and dump the data from memory (correctly formatted)
onto magnetic tape. There are provisions to control how
many channels are sampled, when these channels are sampled,
and when the memory dump is made.

The DAS has an event start input which starts the sampling process in the DAS. When the event start pulse is
received, the converter (A/D) starts digitizing analog signals on the analog inputs. The DAS scans the number of
channels set by the user (in this experiment only one channel, channel zero, is used), at a rate determined by the
sample rate or an external sample rate pulse. The number
of scans made per event start pulse is controlled by the
scans/event which is set by the user. Disabling the scans/
event allows the system to sample continuously.

The analog to digital (A/D) converter converts an
analog signal to 12 digital bits, which include the sign bit.
There are four additional bits. These 16 bits are broken
into two 8-bit characters which make up a word. The memory
has 1K (1024) 8-bit locations, so that 512 2-character words
can be written into memory. Care must be taken not to let

the DAS put more than 512 2-bit words into memory, before
starting to write onto magnetic tape. Once the DAS starts
writing on magnetic tape the DAS can then continue to write
into memory, starting at memory locations whose contents
have been removed.

The memory dump is initiated when a block has been
filled. A block is made up of a number of words, the number
being controlled by the user with the block length switch
on the DAS. A block of 1 corresponds to one 8-bit character.
So, to write a single 16-bit (2 character) word on tape, a
block length of 2 must be used. This block length becomes
important in formatting the read statement later.

To control the DAS, an event start pulse and a scaled
(±10V full scale) analog signal are needed. These two signals are provided from the interface unit, which is the subject of the next chapter.

CHAPTER II

INTERFACE HARDWARE

The purpose of the interface unit is to accept output
signals from the sampling oscilloscope and provide appropriate inputs to the DAS. A block diagram of the interface
unit is shown in Fig. 2.1. The interface unit is designed
to use four inputs from the sampling oscilloscope: the
vertical and horizontal deflection voltages; the vertical
blanking pulses; and a start pulse. The output signals to
the DAS are the gated event start pulses and a scaled
analog signal. The interface unit conditions the outputs
of the sampling oscilloscope in order to control the DAS
and to transfer the information from one sweep of the sampling oscilloscope to the DAS.

The interrelationship of the vertical and horizontal
deflection voltages and the vertical blanking pulses is
critical to the operation of the interface unit. A typical
single sweep showing the dot display, the vertical and horizontal deflection voltages and the vertical blanking pulses
are all illustrated in Fig. 2.2.

The signals from the sampling oscilloscope are obtained
as follows: 1) the vertical and horizontal deflection voltages are available from front panel connections on the

·661
Output
Signals

DAS Input Signals

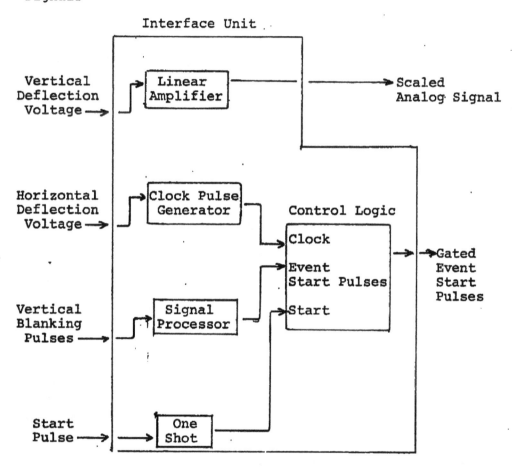

Interface Unit

Vertical
Deflection
Voltage →

Linear
Amplifier

→ Scaled
Analog Signal

Horizontal
Deflection
Voltage →

Clock Pulse
Generator

Control Logic

Clock

Event
Start Pulses

→ Gated
Event
Start
Pulses

Vertical
Blanking
Pulses →

Signal
Processor

Start

Start
Pulse →

One
Shot

Fig. 2.1   Block diagram of the interface unit showing
          overall flow of signals from 661 sampling
          oscilloscope to the data acquisition system.

11

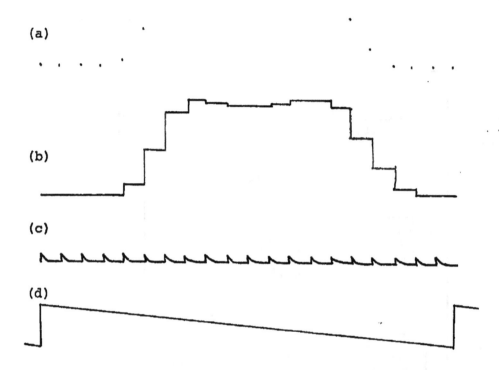

Fig. 2.2   Timing of signals in the sampling oscilloscope:
(a) dot display; (b) vertical deflection
voltage; (c) vertical blanking pulses;
(d) horizontal deflection voltage.

sampling oscilloscope; 2) the start pulse is taken from the single sweep button on the 5T3 timing unit plug in on the sampling oscilloscope. The button is connected internally by the user to a user mounted front panel connector; 3) the vertical blanking pulses are available at a pin on the edge of the trigger and fast ramp board of the 5T3 timing unit. The pin is user connected to the feed-through connector in the sampling oscilloscope and then brought to the back of the sampling oscilloscope. The user mounted connections have been mounted on the 5T3 timing unit serial #001021 and 661 sampling oscilloscope serial #00382.

Both the vertical blanking pulses and the horizontal voltages are processed by the interface unit to produce rectangular pulses having a 5.0V amplitude. The leading edge of the sampling oscilloscope timing signals (vertical blank and horizontal voltages) coincide with the leading edge of the rectangular pulses. The horizontal deflection voltage becomes a clock pulse used in the interface unit. The vertical blanking pulses become the event start pulses for the DAS. The conditioning of the sampling oscilloscope signals is discussed in detail in the following paragraphs, corresponding to the 5 blocks of Fig. 2.1.

The vertical deflection voltage is connected to a high slew rate operational amplifier (LM118) connected in a voltage follower mode as shown in Fig. 2.3. This stage transforms the variable output impedance of the sampling oscilloscope to a small constant impedance. This buffering is done

13

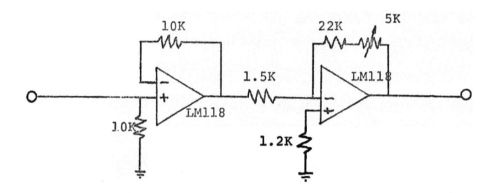

Fig. 2.3 Schematic of the linear amp.

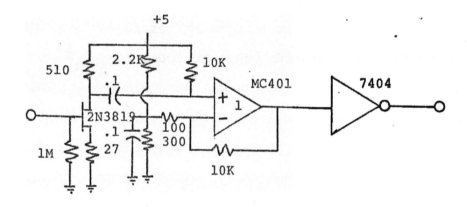

Fig. 2.4 Schematic of the signal processor.

because the gain of following operational amplifier depends
on the source impedance. Since the sampling oscilloscope
output impedance is subject to some variation due to temper-
ature changes, the buffer stage is needed to make the gain
of the linear amplifier (Fig. 2.1) insensitive to these
variations. The gain of the second stage is set to give a
±10.0V output for a full scale vertical deflection, and is
adjustable for calibration. The output of the linear amplifier is connected to channel 0 of the DAS.

The vertical blanking pulse generator provides an output that is small in amplitude (about 250MV into 10MΩ).
The input stage of the signal processor (schematic shown in
Fig. 2.4) is a JFET operated in a common source configuration
which provides 1 MΩ of the input impedance. The drain is
capacitor coupled to the noninverting input of an MC3401
operational amplifier. Advantage is taken of the very fast
turn on time of the operational amplifier to produce a
(4.0V P-P) signal which is capable of driving TTL logic. A
logic inverter is used on the output of the operational
amplifier to produce rectangular pulses which are positive
going. The prime consideration in the signal processor is
to have minimum propagation delay of the leading edge of the
input pulse. The waveforms at various points in the circuit
are shown in Fig. 2.5. The output pulses are the event
start pulses which form the first one of the inputs we have
discussed to the control logic.

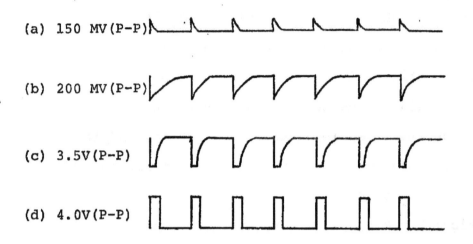

(a) 150 MV (P-P)

(b) 200 MV (P-P)

(c) 3.5V (P-P)

(d) 4.0V (P-P)

Fig. 2.5 Waveforms at various points of the signal
processor (a) gate of the JFET; (b) drain
of JFET; (c) output of op amp; (d) output
of logic.

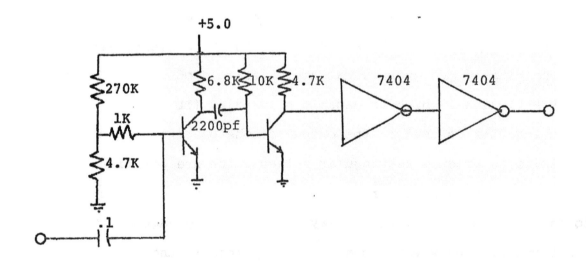

Fig. 2.6 Schematic of the clock pulse generator.

Another input to the control logic is the clock pulse
which is derived from the horizontal deflection voltage.
The schematic for the clock pulse generator is shown in
Fig. 2.6. The clock pulse generator is a grounded emitter
comparator which produces a 20µS pulse. The comparator
fires on the positive going edge of the horizontal deflection voltage. Waveforms of the clock pulse generator are
shown in Fig. 2.7.

The third input to the control logic is the start
pulse. Depressing the single sweep button fires a one-shot
multivibrator which eliminates the effect of contact bounce.
The schematic of the start pulse generator is shown in Fig.
2.8.

The inputs to the control logic (shown in Fig. 2.9)
are the clock pulse, the event start pulses and the start
pulses. The output is a train of gated event start pulses.
The gated event start pulses are present for the duration
of one sweep of the sampling oscilloscope and appear only
after the start button has been depressed. Depressing the
start button sets a set-reset flip-flop (flip-flop 1 of
Fig. 2.9). The flip-flop remains set until the next clock
pulse (the start of the next sweep). On the rise of the
clock pulse, the set flip-flop sets a J-K flip-flop. The
J-K flip-flop remains set until the next pulse clock, at
which time the J-K flip-flop resets. While in the set state,
the J-K flip-flop gates event start pulses to the DAS. In
this manner, the DAS is provided the timing to sample the

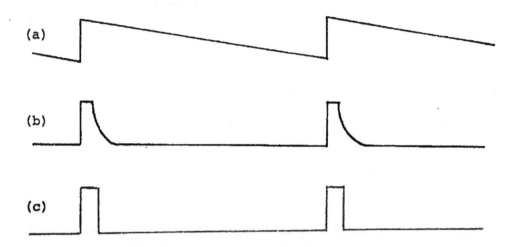

Fig. 2.7 Waveforms from clock pulse generator
(a) horizontal deflection voltage;
(b) output of comparator circuit;
(c) clock output.

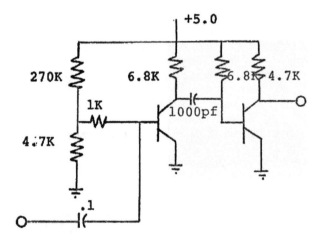

Fig. 2.8 Start pulse generator.

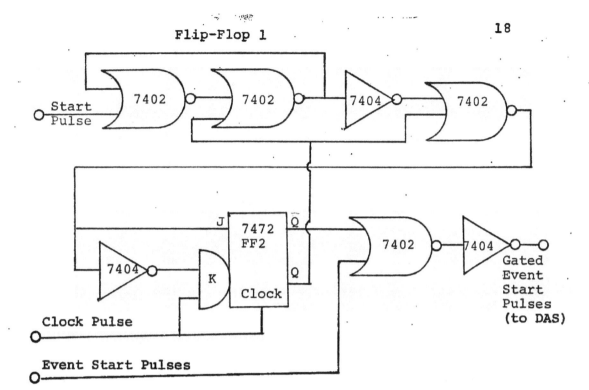

Fig. 2.9 Logic diagram of the control logic.

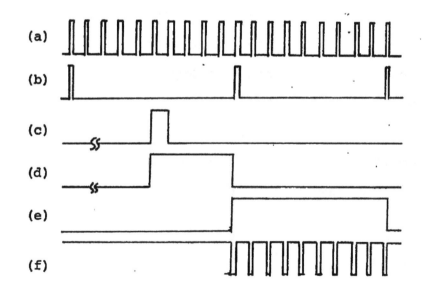

Fig. 2.10 Timing diagram of the control logic
(a) event start pulses from signal
processor; (b) clock pulses from
clock pulse generator; (c) start pulse;
(d) set pulse; (e) gating pulse;
(f) gated event start pulse.

scaled analog signal for one sweep of the sampling oscilloscope. A timing diagram of the control logic is shown in
Fig. 2.10.

All DC voltages required in the interface unit are
generated internally, eliminating the need for external
power supplies. A schematic of the power supply circuits
is shown in Fig. 2.11. The DC voltages generated from 115
VAC are ±15.0V and are adjustable and +5.0V (which cannot
be adjusted). The deviation of the output of the integrated
regulators which supply the DC voltages is specified as
being ±.01% nominal.

The interface unit accepts voltages from the sampling
oscilloscope as input signals. These voltages are condi-
tioned to control the DAS, and provide a scaled analog input
to the DAS. All DC voltages are generated internally. A
complete interface schematic is found in Appendix A.

Once a sweep has been transferred to the DAS, the DAS
writes the digitized analog signal on magnetic tape. The
data on the magnetic tape is the input to a FORTRAN program
which is the subject of the next chapter.

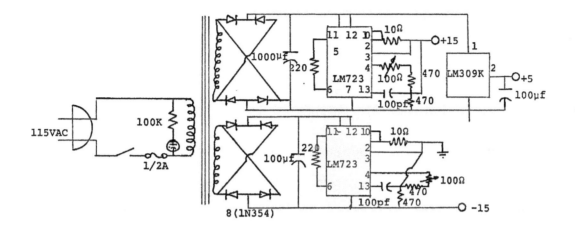

Fig. 2.11 Schematic of power supply.

CHAPTER III

SOFTWARE SUPPORT

The FORTRAN software support designed for the fast
rise time pulse acquisition system reads the magnetic tape
output from the DAS and processes the data. Refer to flow
chart in Fig. 3.1. The waveform is reconstructed, the area
under the curve found, the switching time calculated, and
the results listed, along with a plot of the waveform.
Some of the techniques developed for handling data for the
program have applications for using the DAS in other experiments. These techniques are discussed in some detail below.

The DAS writes the output data with a Precision Instruments model 1209 digital recorder/reproducer (1209) on half
inch computer grade magnetic tape. The 1209 recorder
accepts 8-bit data characters in either binary or binary
coded decimal form. The DAS displays the data being written
in a hexadecimal representation of the binary data.

Once the tape has been written, it is possible to get
a hexadecimal dump of the data on the tape by using the IBM
utility program IEBPTPCH. The Job Control Language (JCL)
for using this utility program is listed in Appendix B.

At the time this software was being developed the A/D
converter in the DAS was inoperative and the manual data

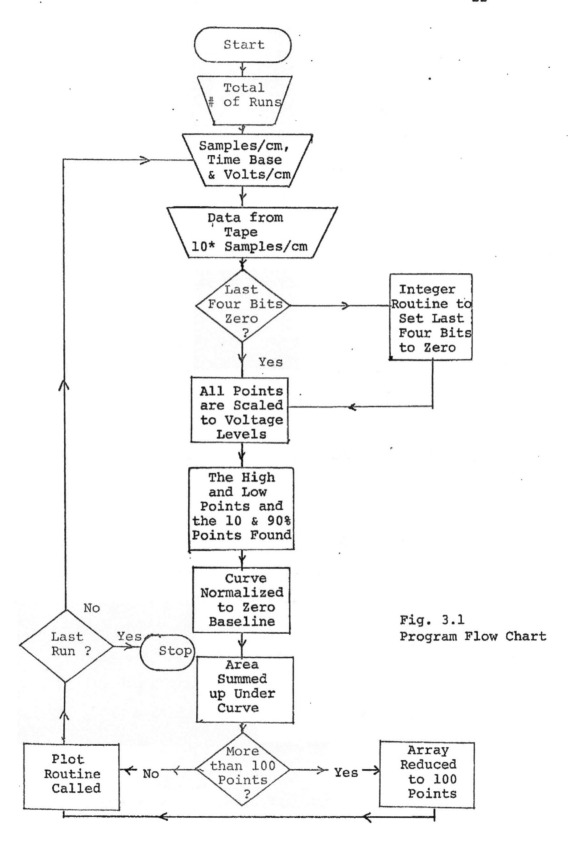

Fig. 3.1
Program Flow Chart

input of the DAS was utilized for writing a trial tape.
Numbers were chosen that were representative of a typical
waveform. The numbers used are listed in Table 1. The
results of a hexadecimal dump are shown in Fig. 3.2.

The discussion that follows is a description of the
main program developed for this project and the discussion
follows the logic of the flow chart on Fig. 3.1.

The problem of reading the tape into a FORTRAN program
was solved by using an A2 (half word) format. Since a
block length of 20 had been used, it was possible to use a
10A2 format. The variable that the data was read into was
specified to be integer *2 (a nonstandard size). Specifying
the variable to be integer *2 means the integer variable
contains the integer representation of the data read in and
contains 16 bits. A 2-character word from the DAS contains
16 bits. An implied DO loop reads the entire record.

At this point all the data is in a FORTRAN array and
ready to be processed. The program listed in Appendix C
read in all the data found in Fig. 3.2 and wrote this data
in an integer format. The results are listed in Fig. 3.3.

Thus by knowing how many data points are on the tape
(which can be found from a hexadecimal dump if necessary),
it is a simple matter to enter data to a FORTRAN program
from a magnetic tape by using only FORTRAN statements.

Earlier it was mentioned that the variable would con-
tain 16 bits. The A/D converter converts an analog signal
to a 12-bit number. The last four bits are from a source

TABLE 1

DATA ENTERED TO THE DAS THROUGH MANUAL DATA SWITCHES

Number of Times Characters Were Entered	Hexadecimal Data
10	FFF0
1	EFF0
1	DFF0
1	CFF0
1	BFF0
1	AFF0
2	9FF0
1	8FF0
1	8OF0
1	8000
11	8FF0
1	9FF0
1	AFF0
1	BFF0
1	CFF0
1	DFF0
1	E000
1	EOF0
1	EFF0
11	FFF0

```
FFFOFFFO   FFFOFFFO   FFFOFFFO   FFFOFFFO   FFFOFFFO*
FFFODFFO   CFFOBFFO   AFFO9FFO   9FFOBFFO   80F09000*
BFFOBFFO   8FFOBFFO   8FFOBFFO   8FFO8FFO   8FFO8FFO*
BFFO9FFO   AFFOBFFO   CFFODFFO   E000F0F0   EFFOFFFO*
FFFOFFFO   FFFOFFFO   FFFOFFFO   FFFOFFFO   FFFOFFFO*
```

Fig. 3.2 Hexadecimal Dump of data entered on tape.
The asterisk denotes the end of record.

```
=16       =16       =16       =16       =16       =16       =16       =16       =16       =16
=4112     =8208     =12304    =16400    =20496    =24592    =24592    =28688    =32528    =32768
=28688    =28688    =28688    =28688    =28688    =28688    =28688    =28688    =28688    =28688
=28688    =24592    =20496    =16400    =12304    =8208     =8192     =7952     =4112     =16
=16       =16       =16       =16       =16       =16       =16       =16       =16       =16
```

Fig. 3.3 FORTRAN interpretation of data entered on tape.
The hexadecimal dump is written in 5 32-bit words
per record (line). The tape is written with 16-bit
words (1/2 words) and read with half word variables.
This gives the ten integers per line shown.

other than the A/D (this depends on the machine configuration).
The first task is to test the last four bits for 0. This can
be done in several ways, one of which is to divide the number
by 16 in integer arithmetic. Multiplying the quotient by
16 should yield the original number. If the number is not
divisible evenly by 16, one or more of the last 4 bits was
not 0, and it is a straightforward process to test and see
which one was not 0.

The routine chosen is to subtract successively numbers
from 1 to 15 and test each case. When the number is evenly
divisible by 16, the last 4 bits are 0.

Once the last 4 bits test for 0, the number is scaled,
inverted (the hardware inverts the signal) and multiplied
by the voltage scale. The data are now in the form of
equivalent voltages. The array contains numbers which re-
present voltages seen on the oscilloscope, and the array is
ready for further processing.

The program finds the high and low points and then finds
the 10% and 90% amplitude points. From 10% and 90% points,
the program can calculate the switching time, defined as
the time it takes for the voltage to go from the 10% to
the 90% points. The low point is subtracted from all points
to normalize the waveform to a 0.0V baseline. The low
point becomes the DC offset. Using trapezoidal integration
the area under the curve is summed up. The array is now
ready to set up for plotting.

A special plot routine was designed for the system. The plot routine prints out an 8 square by 10 square grid (representing the oscilloscope grid) and plots the waveform, using 100 points. If the array was larger than 100 points, the array is reduced to 100 points. The page with the wave-form plot is titled with the run number, the voltage and time scales. Switching time, area, DC offset and samples/cm are listed just below the grid. All data pertaining to one run are listed on one page, and there are enough lines left to print out any additional parameters or conditions the user might desire.

A flow chart of the program is shown in Fig. 3.1.

This chapter has described the development and logic flow of the FORTRAN support software used to read and process the magnetic tape output of the DAS. Complete main program and plot subroutine listings are in Appendix D. The output from the data shown in Fig. 3.2 and Fig. 3.3 is shown in Fig. 3.4.

28

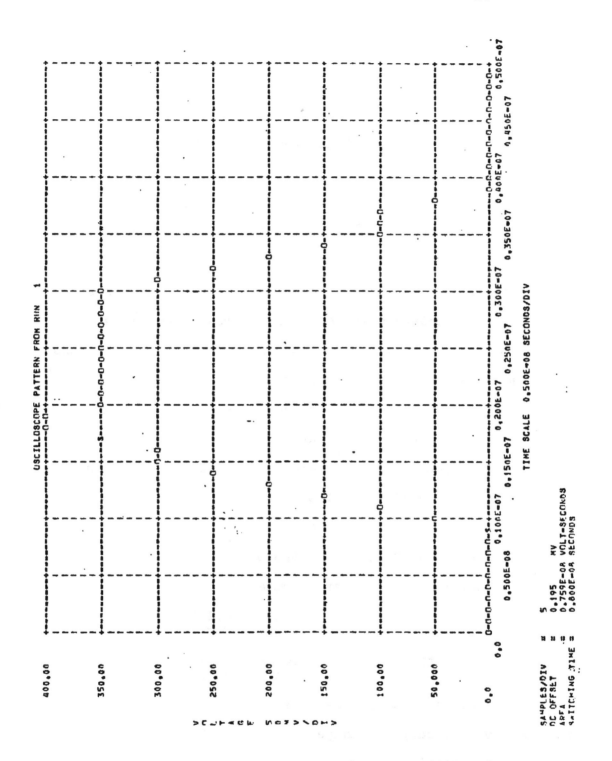

Fig. 3.4 Output of main program using data found in Table I.
Sample of FORTRAN deck is found in Appendix D.

CHAPTER IV

USING THE FAST RISE TIME PULSE DATA ACQUISITION SYSTEM

This chapter will give the user the information he needs to connect all the parts of the system and make the system work.

The system described is comprised of three pieces of equipment and software support. The hardware consists of a Tektronix 661 sampling oscilloscope, an interface unit and a Datacom 8015 data acquisition system.

The sampling oscilloscope should be turned on and allowed to warm up for 30 minutes so that drift is minimized. The settings on the sampling oscilloscope and the plug in units are listed below.

Type 661

Horizontal Display	Sweep Magnifier X1
Position and Vernier	Centered
Amplitude/Time Calibrator	1000MV Amplitude, 1μSec/Cycle
Intensity	Set for normal trace brightness
Focus and Astigmatism	Centered

It may be necessary to change the CRT settings for proper focus and intensity.

Type 4S3 Plug In

Mode	A
'A' Position	Midrange
'A' Smoothing	Clockwise
'A' Millivolts/Cm	200
'A' Variable	Calibrated (at detent)
Triggering	A-AC
DC Offset	Set to zero with voltmeter connected to offset monitor jack (only rough adjustment need be made as another final adjustment is made with the interface connected)

Other controls may be in any position.

Type 5T3

EQUIVALENT TIME/CM	.2µSEC (MAGNIFIER engaged with TIME POSITION RANGE)
Equivalent Time/Cm VARIABLE	CAL (counterclockwise at detent)
Equivalent Time SAMPLES/CM	Midrange (20 for SN 101-1999)
TIME POSITION	Clockwise
Time Position FINE	Centered
SWEEP MODE	NORM
REAL TIME/CM	.5mSEC
TRIG LEVEL	Clockwise
STABILITY OR UHF SYNC	Clockwise
TRIG SOURCE	FREE RUN
SLOPE	+

This setup will produce a free running trace on the CRT.

At this point the interface unit can be connected. The

side of the interface labelled "input" has four leads which
are individually labelled. The start lead is plugged into
the 5T3 start jack (located below and to the right of the
single sweep start button). The vertical signal input is
plugged into the appropriate vertical signal output jack
(there are two, A and B. The setup given assumes channel A
to be used, however channel B can be used instead). The
horizontal signal input is plugged into the horizontal signal output jack. The vertical blanking input is plugged into the vertical blanking output located on the back of the
sampling oscilloscope (located on the upper left of the back
of the sampling oscilloscope). Plug the interface power
cord in and turn on the "power on" switch. The system is
now ready for calibration.

Adjust the free running trace to the bottom of the grid
on the CRT screen. Monitor the voltage on the analog output of the interface unit. It should be zero volts. If it
is not, adjust the DC offset on the sampling oscilloscope
until the output of the interface is zero. Then position
the trace on the bottom line of the grid. The interface is
now ready to plug into the Datacom 8015 data acquisition
system (DAS). Plug the analog output of the interface unit
into channel 0 of the DAS. Plug the event start lead into
event start on the DAS. Set up the DAS as follows:

DAS Setup

Mode Switch	Auto
Sample Rate	32 (KHz)
Enable/Disable	Enable
Scans/Event	001
Block Length	0200
Char. per Word	2
Display Chan	000
Chan/Scan	001
Memory Load Enable	Off (light off)
Memory Test	Off
Write/Read	Write On
Power	On

Turn on the power to the tape unit, load a tape with a write ring installed on the Precision Instruments tape unit. Depressing the ready button and then the load button advances the tape to the marker on the tape. The BOT advance indicator light should be on; if it is not on, depress the stop button on the tape unit, put the write/ read button in the read position and depress the rewind button on the tape unit. The tape will rewind and turn on the BOT advance light. Depressing the ready button on the tape unit and then the BOT advance button advances the tape to the correct distance from the marker to begin recording data. Put the DAS in the write mode and the system is now ready to begin acquiring data.

Obtain a waveform on the sampling oscilloscope that you wish to record. Depressing the start button transfers one sweep of the sampling oscilloscope to the DAS. (The tape should increment slightly.) Depress the EOF (end of file) at least once and then depress the system reset on the DAS. The system is now ready for another waveform setup.

Data that need to be recorded are: 1) the total number of runs made, 2) the samples/cm for each run, 3) time base (secs/cm), and 4) volts/cm.

The data are entered on cards as follows:

First card: total number of runs made entered as a decimal number anywhere on the card.

Second and subsequent cards (one for each run): the samples/cm entered in an F10.0 format (a decimal number entered anywhere in the first ten columns); time base entered as a decimal or exponential in colums 11-20 (exponential right justified), and volts/cm entered as a decimal or exponential in columns 21-30 (exponential right justified). This data entered behind the FORTRAN deck along with the appropriate JCL will give a plot of the waveform, a listing of scale information, samples/cm, DC offset, area under the curve and the switching time. $ marks are placed on the plot at about the 10 and 90% points.

A listing of an example of the complete deck, along with a sample output is given in Appendix D.

The user should be aware of the fact that the individual pieces of equipment can be operated in many modes and the

modes described in this chapter are simply one way of
operating the system. The user should have enough information to successfully operate the systems in the mode
described.

CHAPTER V

SUMMARY

This thesis has described the development of a data acquisition and processing system for digitizing and analyzing fast rise time pulses.

The system uses a Tektronix 661 sampling oscilloscope to provide analog samples of the fast rise time pulses. A Datacom 8015 data acquisition system digitizes and stores the samples and writes the data on magnetic tape. A FORTRAN program reduces the data to switching time, the area under the curve and a plot of the digitized samples.

A potential difficulty exists in the approach adopted in the implementation of the interface hardware. The gating of the DAS sample and hold amplifier is controlled by the DAS sample rate clock which is free running and not synchronized with the sampling in the 661. The highest DAS sample rate is 32 KHz, which means that a sample is taken randomly within an interval of 31.25μsec maximum. Should this randomness be a problem, the interface can be modified in the following manner: first, use the $\overline{Q}$ of flip-flop 2 (the J-K flip-flop) as an event start pulse; second, connect the signal which was the gated event start pulse to the external sample rate input; third, set the sample rate to external;

35

fourth, disable the scans/event. The sampling by the DAS
will then occur at fixed intervals after the gated event
start pulses (the new external sample rate) go negative.
This modification was not made in the development in order
to keep the connections as simple as possible.

The result of this development effort is a complete
system that can sample and display fast rise time pulses.
The display is a hard copy with a listing of parameters and
the results of several computations printed on a single
sheet.

APPENDIX A - SCHEMATIC OF INTERFACE UNIT

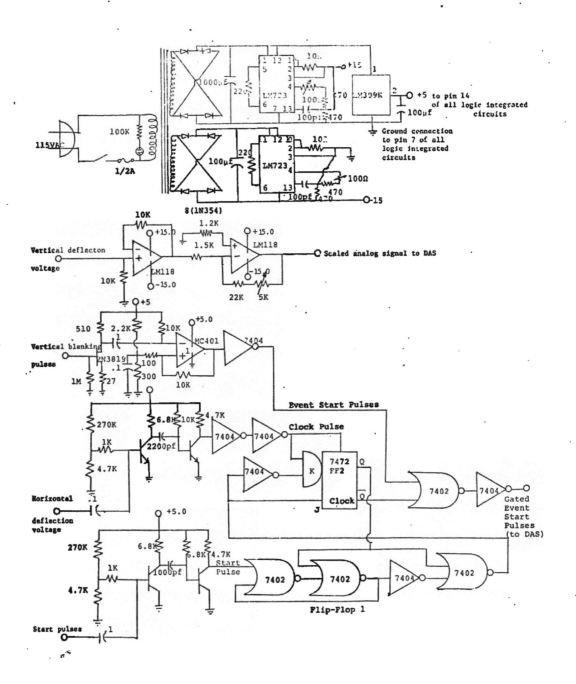

APPENDIX B - JOB CONTROL LANGUAGE DECK
TO OBTAIN A HEXADECIMAL DUMP
FROM A 9-TRACK TAPE NAMED
FEATRE

```
// EXEC PGM=IEBPTPCH
//SYSPRINT CD SYSOUT=A
//SYSUT1 DC UNIT=TAPE9,VOL=SER=FEATRE,LABEL=(1,NL),
//       DCB=(RECFM=U,BLKSIZE=10C00),DISP=(OLD,KEEP)
//SYSUT2 CC SYSCUT=A
//SYSIN CD *
 PRINT TCTCCNV=XE,STOPAFT=21
```

APPENDIX C - FORTRAN PROGRAM USED TO READ
A TAPE NAMED <u>FEATRE</u> TO OBTAIN
DATA FOUND IN FIG. 3.3

```
//  EXEC  F4GCXS
//FCRT.SYSIN CC *
      INTEGER*2 K
      DIMENSICN K(10)
    1 FORMAT(10A2)
    2 FCRMAT(10I10)
      DO 10 I=1,5
      READ(1,1)(K(J),J=1,10)
      WRITE(6,2)(K(J),J=1,10)
   10 CONTINUE
      STOP
      END
//GC.FTO1F001 CD UNIT=(TAPE9,,DEFER),VOL=SER=FEATRE,DSN=X,
//  LABEL=(1,NL,,IN),DCB=(RECFM=U,BLKSIZE=10000,LRECL=10000),
//  DISP=OLC
```

APPENDIX D - MAIN PROGRAM WITH JCL, PLOT
SUBROUTINE AND SAMPLE DATA.
THIS GIVES THE OUTPUT FOUND
IN FIG. 3.4.

```
//   EXEC   F4GCXS
//FORT.SYSIN DO *
      DIMENSION K(100),Y(100),X(100),Z(100)
      INTEGER*2 K
    1 FORMAT(10A2)
    2 FORMAT(F80.0)
    3 FORMAT(3F10.0)
    4 FORMAT(' ',T4,'AREA',T19,'=',T23,G10.3,' VOLT-SECONDS',
     1/,T4,'SWITCHING TIME',T19,'=',T23,G10.3,' SECONDS')
    5 FORMAT('1')
    6 FORMAT(' ',T4,'DC OFFSET',T19,'=',T23,G10.3,' MV')
    7 FORMAT('0',T4,'SAMPLES/DIV',T19,'=',T21,I4)
      READ(5,2)RUNS
      NRUNS=RUNS
      DO 100 II=1,NRUNS
C     THE PROGRAM SETS UP THE NUMBER OF RUNS TO BE MADE
      M=0
      READ(5,3)SAMPLE,TBASE,VSCALE
C     SAMPLES/CM,TIME BASE(SECS/CM),AND VOLTS/CM ARE READ IN
      NSAMPL=10*SAMPLE
      READ(1,1)(K(I),I=1,NSAMPL)
C     DATA READ IN FROM TAPE IN INTEGER REPRESENTATION OF BINARY
      DO 10 I=1,NSAMPL
      J=K(I)/16
      KK=J*16
      IF(KK.EQ.K(I)) GO TO 12
      DO 11 L=1,15
      J=(K(I)-L)
      KK=16*(J/16)
      IF(KK.NE.J) GO TO 11
      K(I)=J
      GO TO 10
   11 CONTINUE
   12 DUM=K(I)
      Y(I)=(-8.0*VSCALE*DUM)/32767.0
   10 CONTINUE
C     THE FOUR LAST BITS ARE ZERO(ONLY VOLTAGE BITS ARE PRESENT
C     AND THE Y(N) ARRAY CONTAINS THE VOLTAGES SEEN ON THE SCREEN
      SMALL=Y(1)
      RLARGE=Y(1)
      MARKHI=1
      DO 20 I=2,NSAMPL
```

```
      SMALL=Y(I)
   21 CONTINUE
      IF(RLARGE.GT.Y(I)) GO TO 20
      IF(RLARGE.GT.Y(I+1)) M=1
      IF(M.EQ.1) GO TO 20
      RLARGE=Y(I)
      MARKHI=I
   20 CONTINUE
C     THE HIGH AND LOW POINTS HAVE BEEN FOUND
C     THE HIGH POINT IS THE FIRST PEAK
      SWITHI=0.9*RLARGE
      SWITLO=0.1*RLARGE
      LOTIME=1
      NHITIM=1
      DO 30 I=1,MARKHI
      IF(Y(I).GE.SWITLO) GO TO 31
      LOTIME=I
   31 CONTINUE
      IF(Y(I).GE.SWITHI) GO TO 30
      NHITIM=I
   30 CONTINUE
      DIV=NSAMPL
      DIF=NHITIM-LOTIME
      SWTIME=DIF*TBASE*10.0/DIV
C     THE SWITCHING TIME HAS BEEN CALCULATED
      DO 40 I=1,NSAMPL
      X(I)=Y(I)-SMALL
   40 CONTINUE
C     THE CURVE HAS BEEN NORMALIZED TO A ZERO BASELINE
      AREA=0.0
      TIMINC=TBASE*10.0/DIV
      NSAM=NSAMPL-1
      DO 50 I=1,NSAM
      HAVG=(X(I)+X(I+1))/2.0
      AREA=AREA+(HAVG*TIMINC)
   50 CONTINUE
      IF(NSAMPL.LE.100) GO TO 71
      NT=NSAMPL/100
      LOTIME=LOTIME/NT
      NHITIM=NHITIM/NT
      DO 61 I=100
      Y(I)=Y(I*NT)
   61 CONTINUE
C     Y ARRAY HAS BEEN REDUCED TO 100 POINTS FOR PLOTTING
      NSAMPL=NSAMPL/NT
   71 YMAX=(8.0*VSCALE)
      XMAX=10.0*TBASE
      IF(NSAMPL.LT.100) DIV=100./NSAMPL
      DO 70 IA=1,NSAMPL
      VAR=IA-1
      IF(NSAMPL.LT.100) VAR=VAR*DIV
```

```
      Z(IA)=VAR*(TBASE/10.)
  70 CCNTINUE
      VAR=VSCALE*1000.0
      NVCLTS=VAR+1
      CALL PLOT10(Z,X,XMAX,0.0,YMAX,0.0,NSAMPL,NRUNS,
     1NVCLTS,TBASE,LOTIME,NHITIM)
      NS=SAMPLE
      WRITE(6,7)NS
      SMALL=SMALL*1000.0
      WRITE(6,6)SMALL
      WRITE(6,4)AREA,SWTIME
      WRITE(6,5)
 100 CONTINUE
      STOP
      END
      SUBROUTINE PLOT10(X,Y,XMAX,XMIN,YMAX,YMIN,NPTS,NRUN,NVOLTS,
     1TBASE,LOTIME,NHITIM)
      REAL*4 X(NPTS),Y(NPTS),XSC(11),SPAC
      INTEGER TITLE(20),LABEL(20),NUMBER(10)
      LOGICAL*1 SP,SPACE,DIV,BAR,MINUS,PLUS,$PT,LINE(101),
     1          SYMB(2)
      INTEGER*4 YTITLE(51),VERT(16),SPA
      DATA SPACE/' '/,BAR/' '/,MINUS/'-'/,PLUS/'+'/,SPA/' '/,
     1          SYMB/'O','$'/
      DATA VERT/'V','O','L','T','A','G','E',' ',' ',' ','M','V',
     1          '/','D','I','V'/,SPAC/' '/
      DATA NUMBER/'0','1','2','3','4','5','6','7','8','9'/
      DO 113 IC=1,51
      YTITLE(IC)=SPA
 113 CCNTINUE
      DO 10 I=1,NPTS
  10 CONTINUE
      DO 112 IB=1,16
      YTITLE(IB+16)=VERT(IB)
 112 CONTINUE
      NVAR1=NVOLTS/100
      IF(NVAR1.NE.0) YTITLE(24)=NUMBER(NVAR1+1)
      NTEMP=NVCLTS-(NVAR1*100)
      NVAR2=NTEMP/10
      IF(NVAR2.NE.0) YTITLE(25)=NUMBER(NVAR2+1)
      NVAR3=NTEMP-(NVAR2*10)
      YTITLE(26)=NUMBER(NVAR3+1)
      WRITE(6,120)NRUN
      XR = XMAX - XMIN
      YR = YMAX - YMIN
      RYS = 0.0
      IYT = 50
      DO 70 I3 = 1,9
      DO 70 I4 = 1,6
      SP = SPACE
      DIV = BAR
```

```
       IYT = IYT - 1
       IF (I4 .NE. 1) GO TO 30
       SP = MINUS
       DIV = PLUS
   30  K = 0
       DO 40 I5 = 1,11
       K = K + 1
       LINE(K) = DIV
       IF (I5 .EQ. 11) GO TO 40
       DO 41 I6 = 1,9
       K = K + 1
   41  LINE(K) = SP
   40  CONTINUE
       IYTR = 50 - IYT
       $PT = .FALSE.
       IF (I4 .NE. 1) GO TO 50
       $PT = .TRUE.
       YSC =(YMAX - RYS*YR/8.)*1000.
       RYS = RYS + 1.0
   50  DO 60 I7A = 1,NPTS
       IX = 100.*(X(I7A)-XMIN)/XR + 1.49999
       IY = 48.*(Y(I7A)-YMIN)/YR + 1.49999
       IF (IY .NE. IYT) GO TO 60
       IF((IX .LT. 1) .OR. (IX .GT. 101)) GO TO 60
       LINE(IX) = SYMB(1)
       IF((I7A.EQ.NHITIM).OR.(I7A.EQ.LOTIME)) LINE(IX)=SYMB(2)
   60  CONTINUE
       IF($PT) WRITE(6,1000) YTITLE(IYTR),YSC,(LINE(II),II=1,101)
       IF(.NOT.$PT) WRITE(6,1100) YTITLE(IYTR),(LINE(II),II=1,101)
       IF(I3 .EQ. 9) GO TO 80
   70  CONTINUE
   80  RXS = 0.0
       DO 90 I8 = 1,11
       XSC(I8) = XMIN + RXS*XR/10.
   90  RXS = RXS + 1.0
       WRITE(6,1200) (XSC(II),II=1,11,2),(XSC(II),II=2,11,2)
       WRITE(6,130)TBASE
  100  FORMAT(20A4)
  110  FORMAT(51A1)
  120  FORMAT('1',/48X,'OSCILLOSCOPE PATTERN FROM RUN ',I3)
  130  FORMAT(/48X,'TIME SCALE ',G10.3,' SECONDS/DIV')
 1000  FORMAT(3X,A1,2X,G12.5,1X,101A1)
 1100  FORMAT(3X,A1,15X,101A1)
 1200  FORMAT(4X,6G20.3/14X,5G20.3)
       RETURN
       END
//GO.SYSIN DD *
1.
5.                5.0E-9   .05
//GO.FT01F001 DD UNIT=(TAPE9,,DEFER),VOL=SER=FEATRE,DSN=X,
//   LABEL=(1,NL,,IN),DCB=(RECFM=U,BLKSIZE=10000,LRECL=10000),
```

// DISP=OLD

45

OSCILLOSCOPE PATTERN FROM RUN 1

400.00

350.00

300.00

250.00

200.00

150.00

100.00

50.000

0.0

VOLTAGE RESOLUTION

0.0   0.500E-08 0.100E-07 0.150E-07 0.200E-07 0.250E-07 0.300E-07 0.350E-07 0.400E-07 0.450E-07 0.500E-07

TIME SCALE 0.500E-08 SECONDS/DIV

SAMPLES/DIV   =   5
DC OFFSET   =   0.195 MV
AREA   =   0.759E-08 VOLT-SECONDS
SWITCHING TIME =   0.800E-08 SECONDS

LIST OF REFERENCES

1. Dietmeyer, D. L., _Logic Design of Digital Systems_, Allyn and Bacon, Inc., Boston; 1971.

2. Millman, J. and Taub, H., _Pulse, Digital and Switching Waveforms_, McGraw-Hill Book Co., Inc., New York; 1965.

3. Vickers, F. D., _Fortran IV, A. Modern Approach_, Holt, Rinehart and Winston, Inc., New York; 1970.

4. "Instruction Manual for Data Acquisition System Model 8015," Datacom, Inc., 40 Lincoln Drive, Fort Walton Beach, Florida.

5. "PI-1207, PI-1209, PI-1209/CRC Digital Recorder/ Reproducer Instruction Manual," Precision Instruments Company, 3170 Porter Drive, Palo Alto, California, Dec. 1969.

6. "Type 4S3 Sampling-Probe Dual-Trace Unit Instruction Manual," Tektronix, Inc., S. W. Millikan Way, P. O. Box 500, Beaverton, Oregon, 1966.

7. "Type 5T3 Timing Unit Instruction Manual," Tektronix, Inc., S.W. Millikan Way, P. O. Box 500, Beaverton, Oregon, 1965.

8. "Type 661 Sampling Oscilloscope Instruction Manual," Tektronix, Inc., S.W. Millikan Way, P. O. Box 500, Beaverton, Oregon, 1965.

BIOGRAPHICAL SKETCH

Peter Tappen Fairchild was born September 24, 1943, at New York City, New York. He spent his childhood in South America, returning to the United States in 1956 for his secondary education. He joined the United States Navy in October, 1960, and was honorably discharged from active duty in August, 1964. He graduated from Central Florida Junior College in May, 1966, and attended the University of Florida and Florida Atlantic University. In March, 1971, he joined the General Systems Division of the IBM Corporation at Boca Raton, Florida, as a student engineer working in test engineering designing test equipment for logic circuits. He returned to the University of Florida in March, 1971, where he received the degree of Bachelor of Science in Electrical Engineering in August, 1972. From September, 1972, until the present time he has worked as a Graduate Teaching Assistant in the Department of Electrical Engineering, University of Florida, while pursuing the degree of Master of Engineering.

He is a member of Eta Kappa Nu and the Institute of Electrical and Electronics Engineers.

He is married to the former Cynthia Ann Groves of Ocala, Florida, and has a son, Charles David Fairchild.

I certify that I have read this study and that in my opinion it conforms to acceptable standards of scholarly presentation and is fully adequate, in scope and quality, as a thesis for the degree of Master of Engineering.

J. K. Watson, Chairman
Associate Professor of Electrical Engineering

I certify that I have read this study and that in my opinion it conforms to acceptable standards of scholarly presentation and is fully adequate, in scope and quality, as a thesis for the degree of Master of Engineering.

A. H. Paige
Associate Professor of Electrical Engineering

This thesis was submitted to the Dean of the College of Engineering and to the Graduate Council, and was accepted as partial fulfillment of the requirements for the degree of Master of Engineering.

June, 1973

Dean, College of Engineering

Dean, Graduate School

www.ingramcontent.com/pod-product-compliance
Lightning Source LLC
Chambersburg PA
CBHW060505060326
40689CB00020B/4641